Happy Healthy Teachers Matter

34 Well-Being Tips and Inspiration for Self-Care

by Karen Tui Boyes

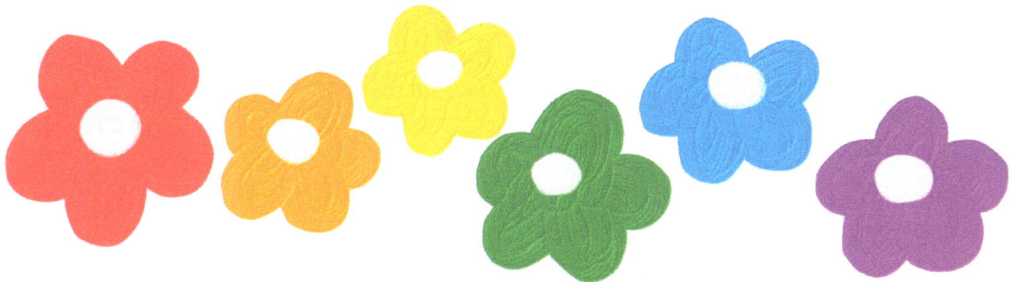

Published by Spectrum Education Limited
Lower Hutt, New Zealand
info@spectrumeducation.com

ISBN 978-0-9951314-6-0

Copyright © Spectrum Education 2023
            © Karen Tui Boyes 2023

Designed and typeset by Spectrum Education, New Zealand

This book contains images from
www.canva.com
Mandala on page 36 drawn by Anna Oosterkamp

To all the educators who tirelessly strive to create a better future for their students, this book is dedicated to you.
It's time to look after YOU!

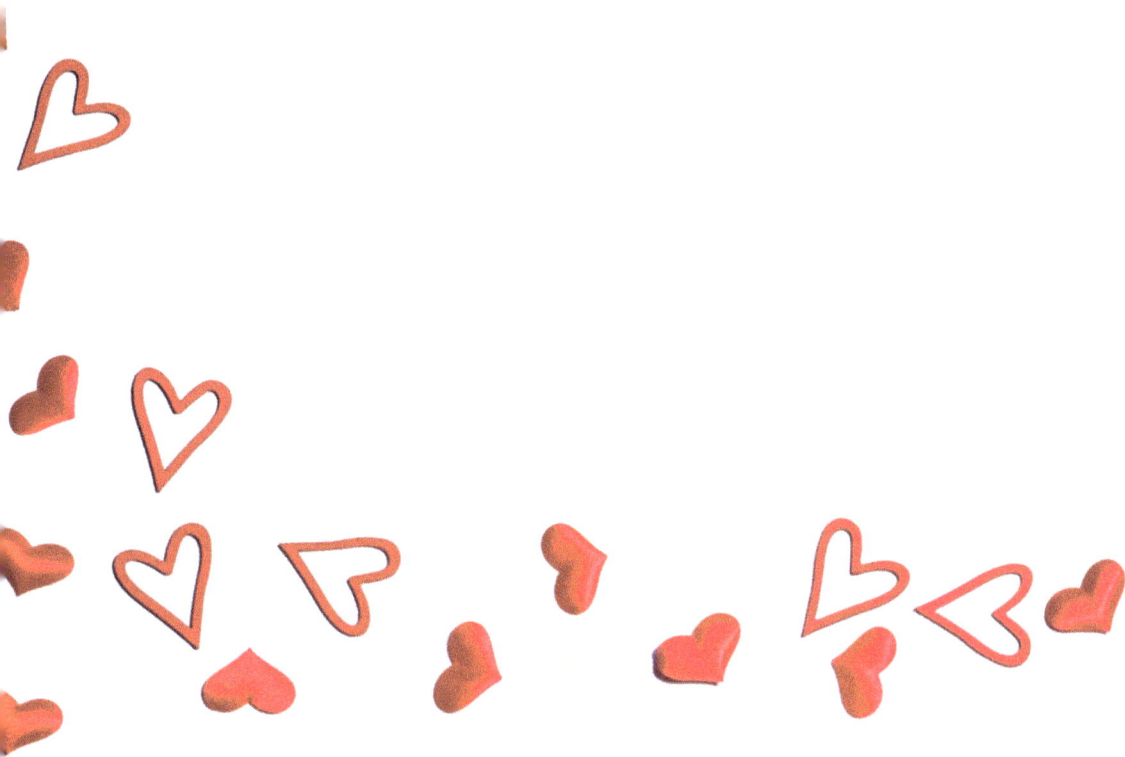

A note from Karen

May this book serve as a reminder that your own well-being is just as important as the well-being of your students, and that by taking care of yourself, you are also taking care of those around you.

Your unwavering commitment to shaping the minds of the next generation is truly inspiring, and I recognise the tremendous effort that goes into making a positive impact on the lives of your students every day.

This book is dedicated to supporting you in taking care of yourself so that you can continue to give your all to your students and your community.

Thank you for all that you do, and for being the change we wish to see in the world.

with rainbow sunshine love,

Karen Tui Boyes
www.karentuiboyes.com
www.spectrumeducation.com

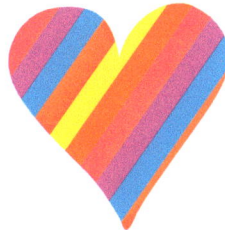

"Time is a precious thing.
Never waste it."

Tip #1: Avoid falling down the rabbit hole...

When looking for ideas on Pinterest and websites - find an idea you can use and stop browsing. Spending hours searching for a 'better' idea is often fruitless and usually a waste of time!

What makes you smile?

1. _____

2. _____

3. _____

4. _____

5. _____

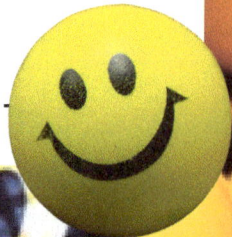

Tip# 2:

Put a smile on your dial

A smile spurs a powerful chemical reaction in the brain that can make you feel happier. Science has shown that the mere act of smiling can lift your mood, lower stress, boost your immune system and possibly even prolong your life.

Setting boundaries is your responsibility. People will continue to do what you allow. You get to decide what is and what isn't allowed in your life.

Tip# 3: Create clear email boundaries...

Create an auto-responder to communicate your working hours and expectations clearly.

"Please note that I check my emails between the hours of 8:15am and 5:00pm Monday to Friday. I will endeavour to respond to your email within 48 hours."

"Morning is an important time of day. Because how you spend your morning can often tell you what kind of day you are going to have."

- Daniel Handler

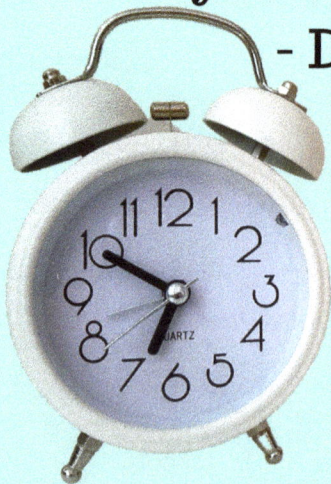

Tip #4: Your morning routine

Start your day with a routine that will help set you up for a great day. Choose something you enjoy: yoga, mindfulness, meditation, stretching, exercise, practice deep breathing, read (use a timer), eat a healthy breakfast (brain food), make the bed (feeling of accomplishment), notice the beauty of nature, kiss and hug your loved ones, do daily affirmations, take a morning walk, do one thing that makes you happy (even if you get up 15 mins earlier for it)... The options are abundant.

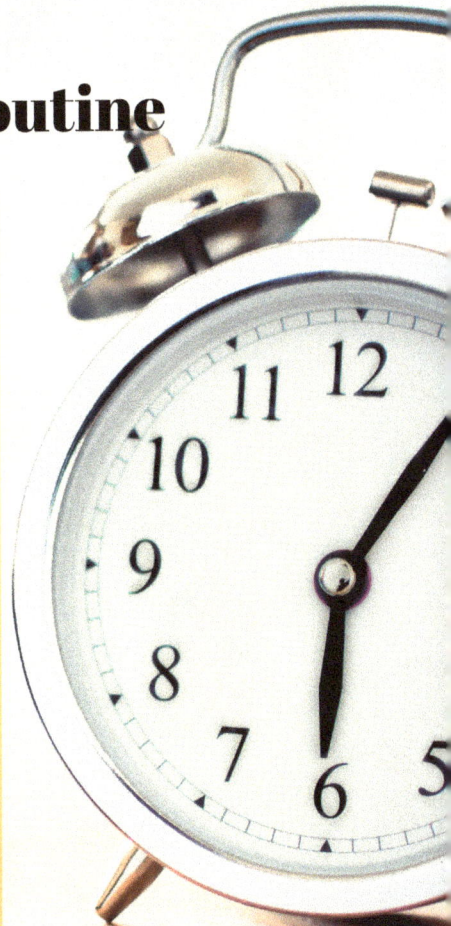

The secret ingredient
is always
LOVE

Tip #5: Batch cook and save time

Once a week spend 1-2 hours in the kitchen and cook & prepare food in bulk. Arrange the food into jars for lunches and dinners. They stay fresher in the glass. Make a triple batch of curry or soup and freeze the extra portions for the nights you get home late or do not have time to cook. This saves so much time and energy during the week.

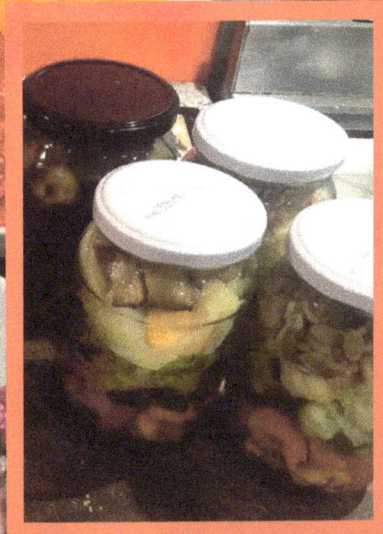

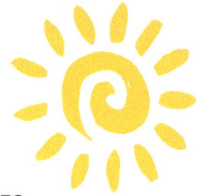

Remember to drink water
and get some sun because
you're basically a houseplant
with more complicated
emotions.

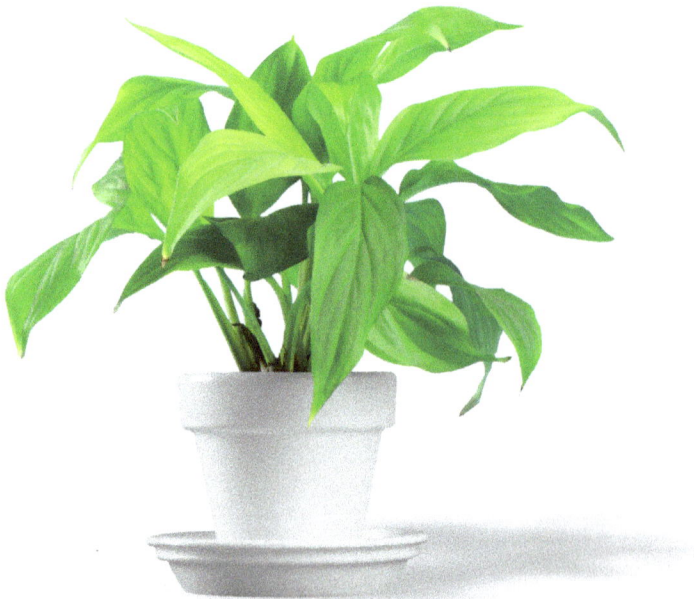

Tip #6: Drink more water...

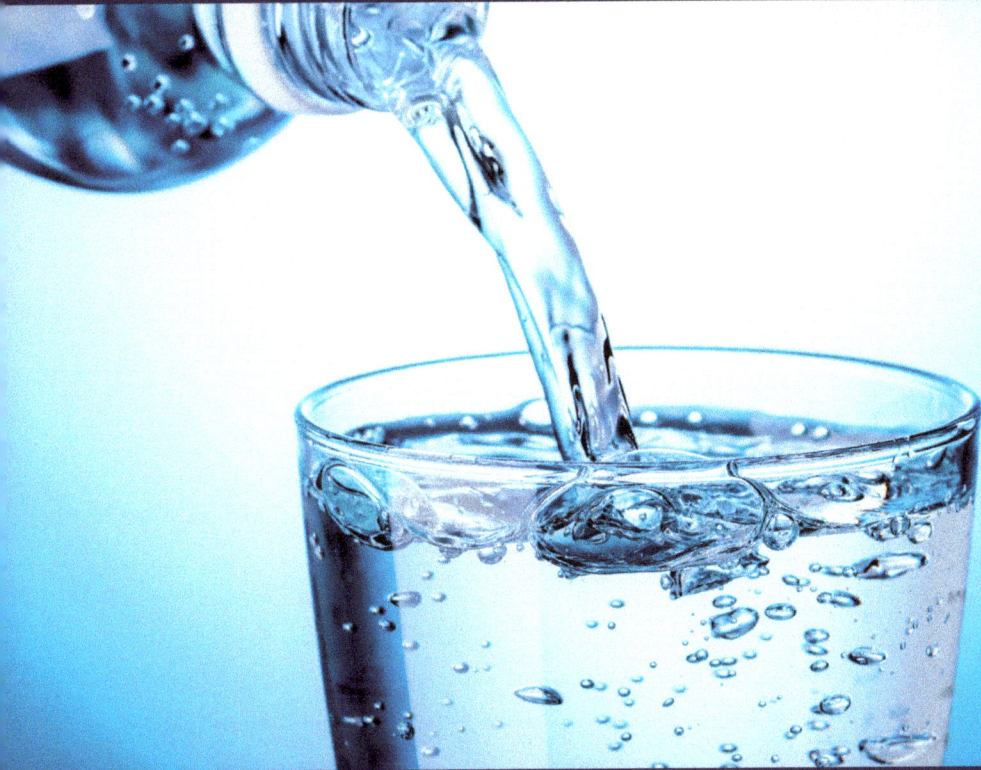

until you've got clear wees...

Rowena McEvoy

My To Do List

1. _____

2. _____

3. _____

4. _____

5. _____

6. _____

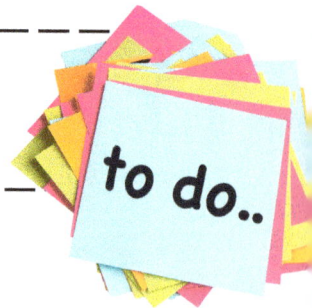

Tip # 7:

To Do List:

- Spend 5 minutes each morning creating a list of your to-do's
- Prioritise
- Start with the most important until it is done
- Move on to the next task...
- Repeat each day...

"For every minute spent organising, an hour is earned."

Tip # 8:

Handle each piece of paper once. Read, sort, file.

You will fall down...
It's the getting up again.
That is the important part

Karen Tui Boyes

Tip #9:

Take your power back

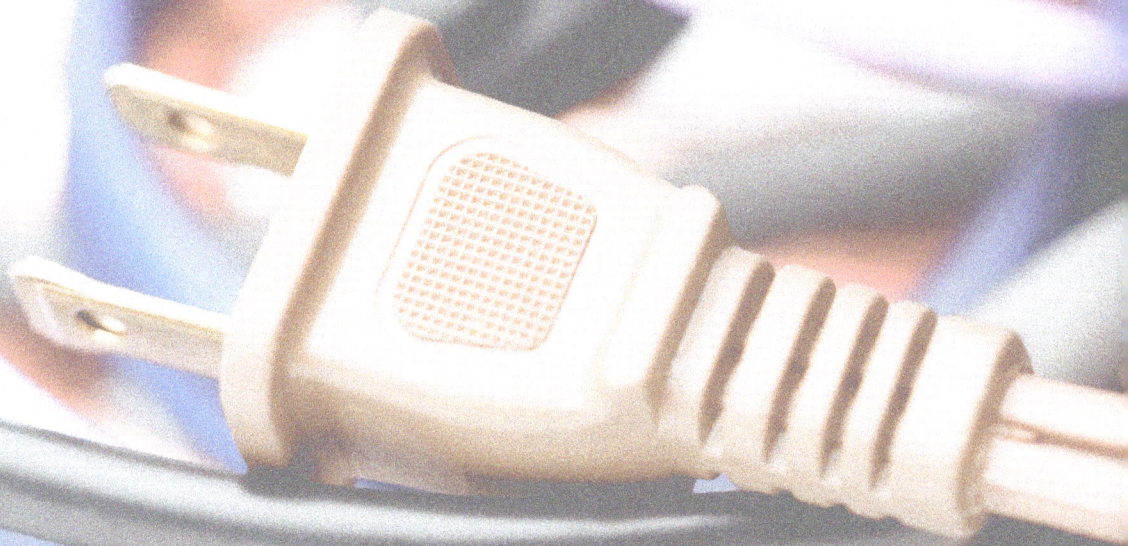

Leave your laptop power cord at school during term time

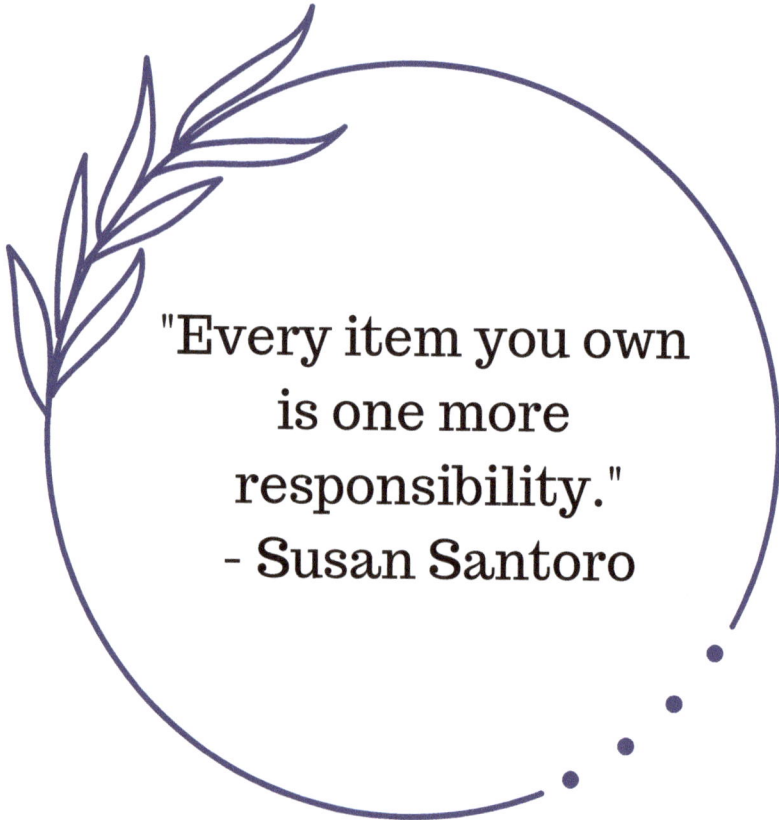

"Every item you own
is one more
responsibility."
- Susan Santoro

Tip #10: Clean out your wardrobe

Decluttering your clothes can reduce stress and increase wellbeing.

Throw out all the clothes that don't fit, you don't like or have not worn in the last 12 months. Give them away to a charity shop, a friend or sell them if you have time. Keeping them often causes extra stress when finding something to wear and pressure to 'have' to lose weight.
Sort your clothes by colour and style to make choosing quick and easy.

Do the hard jobs first.
The easy jobs will take care of
themselves.
-Dale Carnegie

Tip# 11:

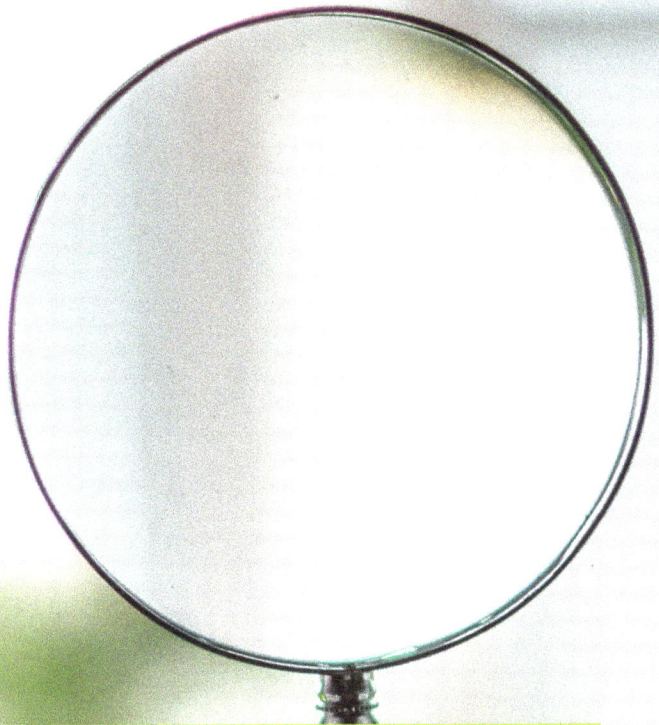

Focus on and talk about being 'productive' every day, rather than being 'busy'.

"A diet rich in fruits and vegetables plays a role in reducing the risk of all the major causes of illness and death."
-Walter Willett

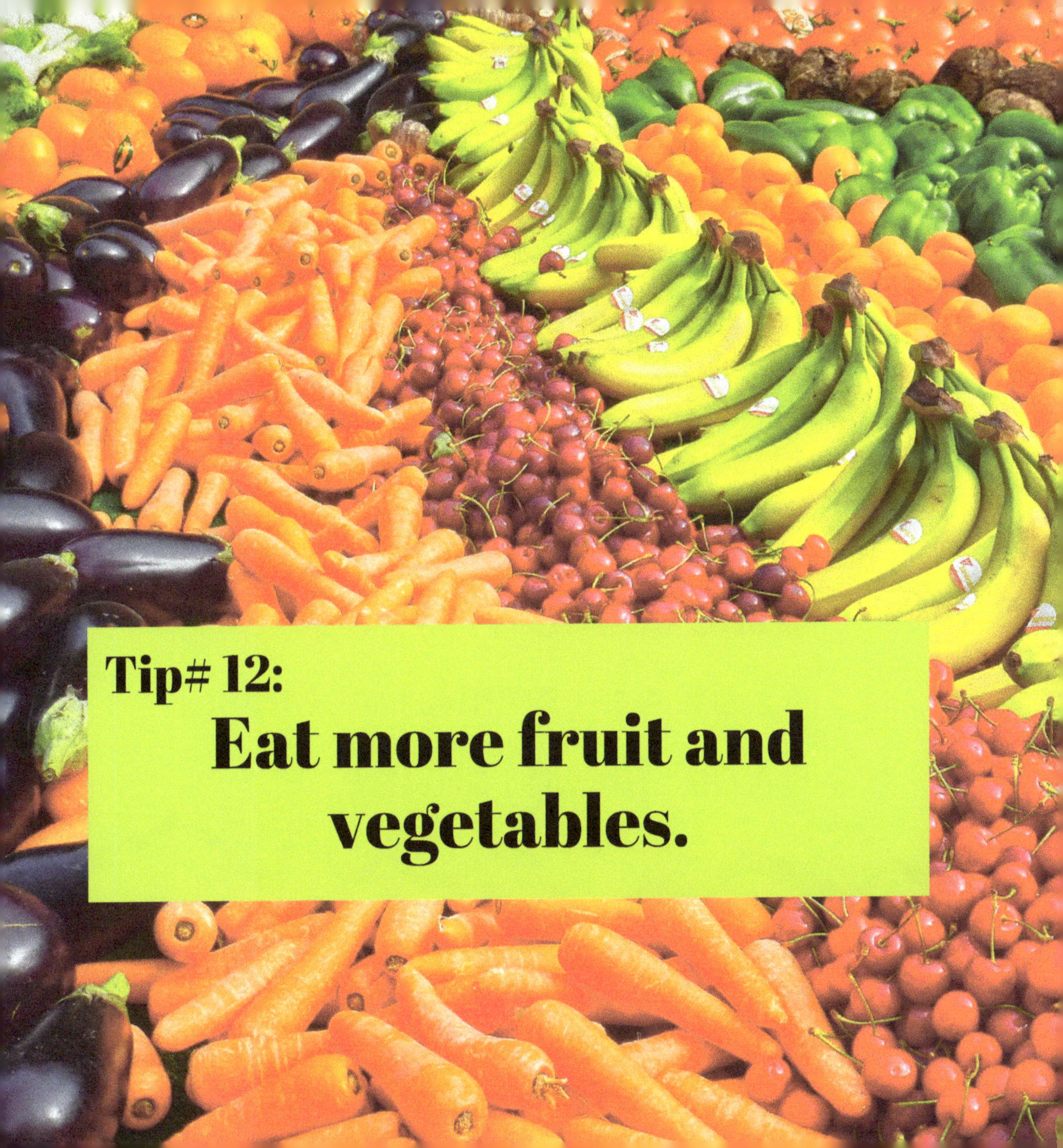

Tip# 12:
Eat more fruit and vegetables.

Things you can control...
- when you ask for help
- what you eat
- the boundaries you set
- how you speak to yourself
- your sleep routine

Tip# 13:

Today I will focus on what I can control

"Change the world by your example, not your opinion."
- Paulo Coelho

Tip# 14: Start a soup or salad club

Club members take turns to prepare different soups or salads to share with the group. By initiating a Salad Club, you can encourage your workmates to eat healthy food, while experimenting with different recipes.

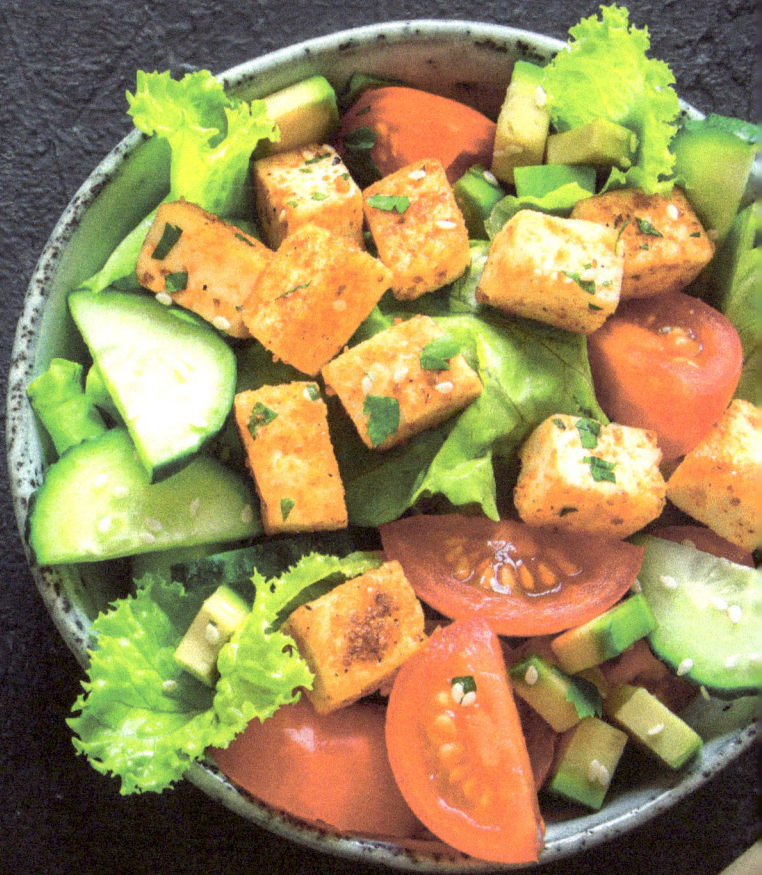

Discipline weighs ounces, while regret weighs TONS.
-Jim Rohn

Tip# 15: Minimise screen time at night

Turn off screens 2-3 hours prior to bedtime to improve your sleep. This includes TV, computers, tablets and phones. If 2-3 hours is too much time, start small and work up to it.

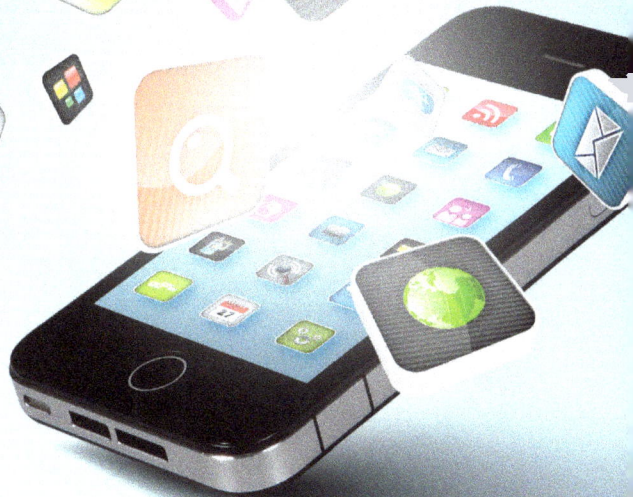

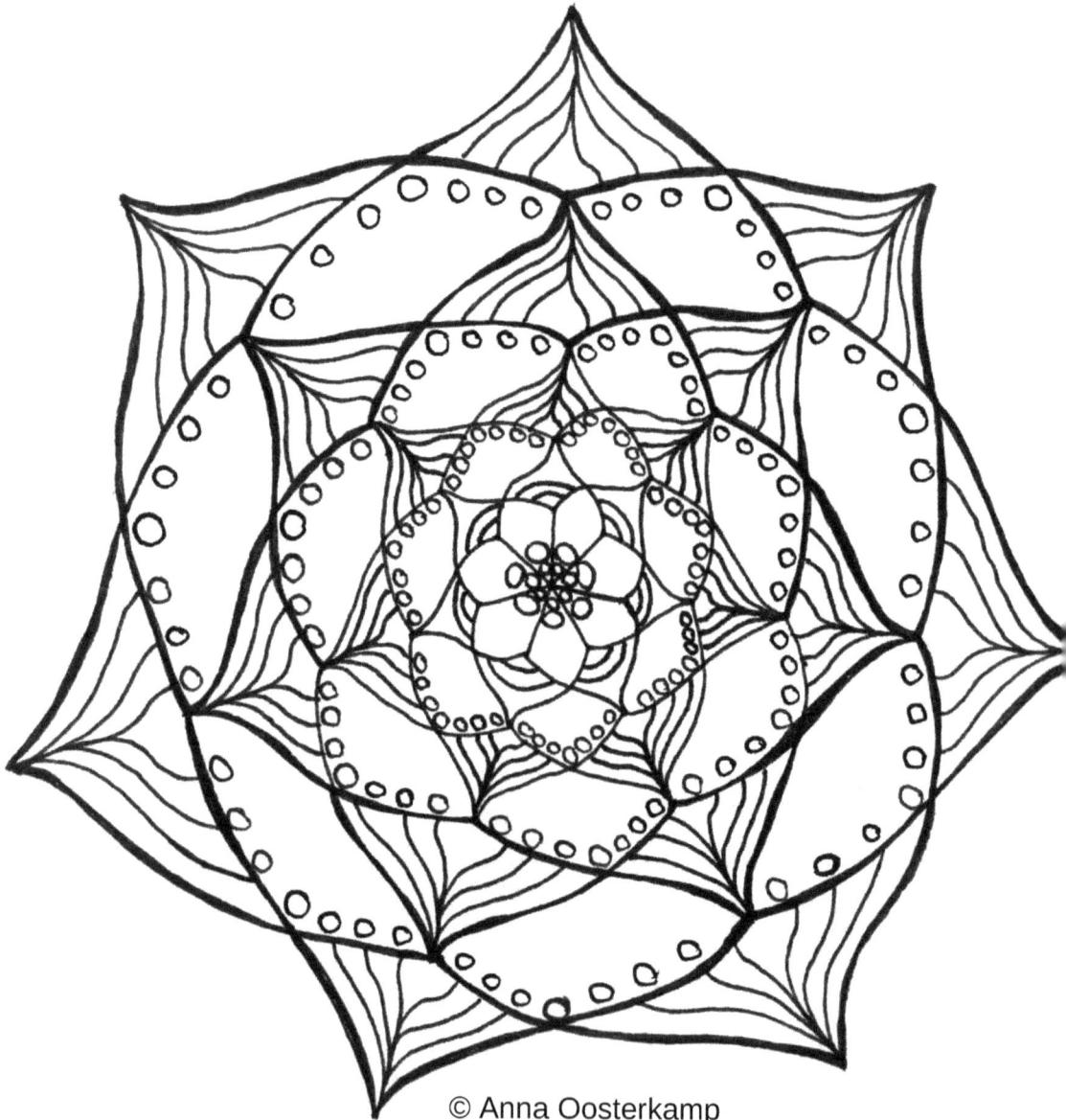

© Anna Oosterkamp

Tip# 16: Do something creative each day

Studies show people who engaged in creative pursuits feel significantly more energetic, enthusiastic, and excited the next day. Creative activities include; drawing, colouring, knitting, gardening, photography, baking, writing, dancing, singing, designing and so much more.

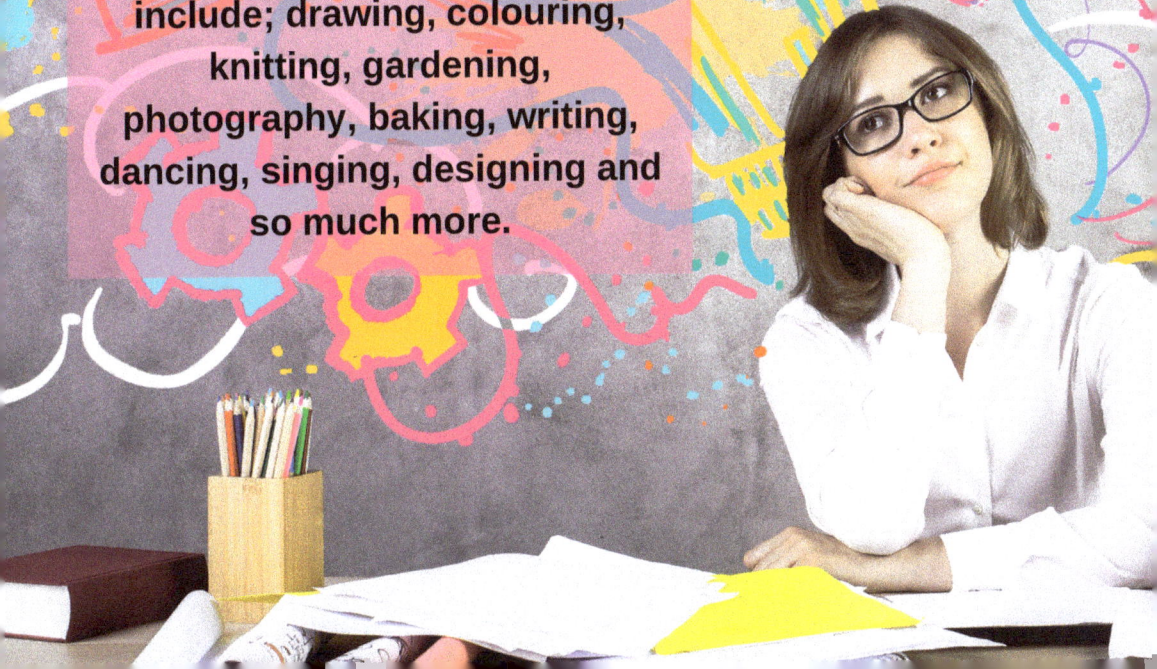

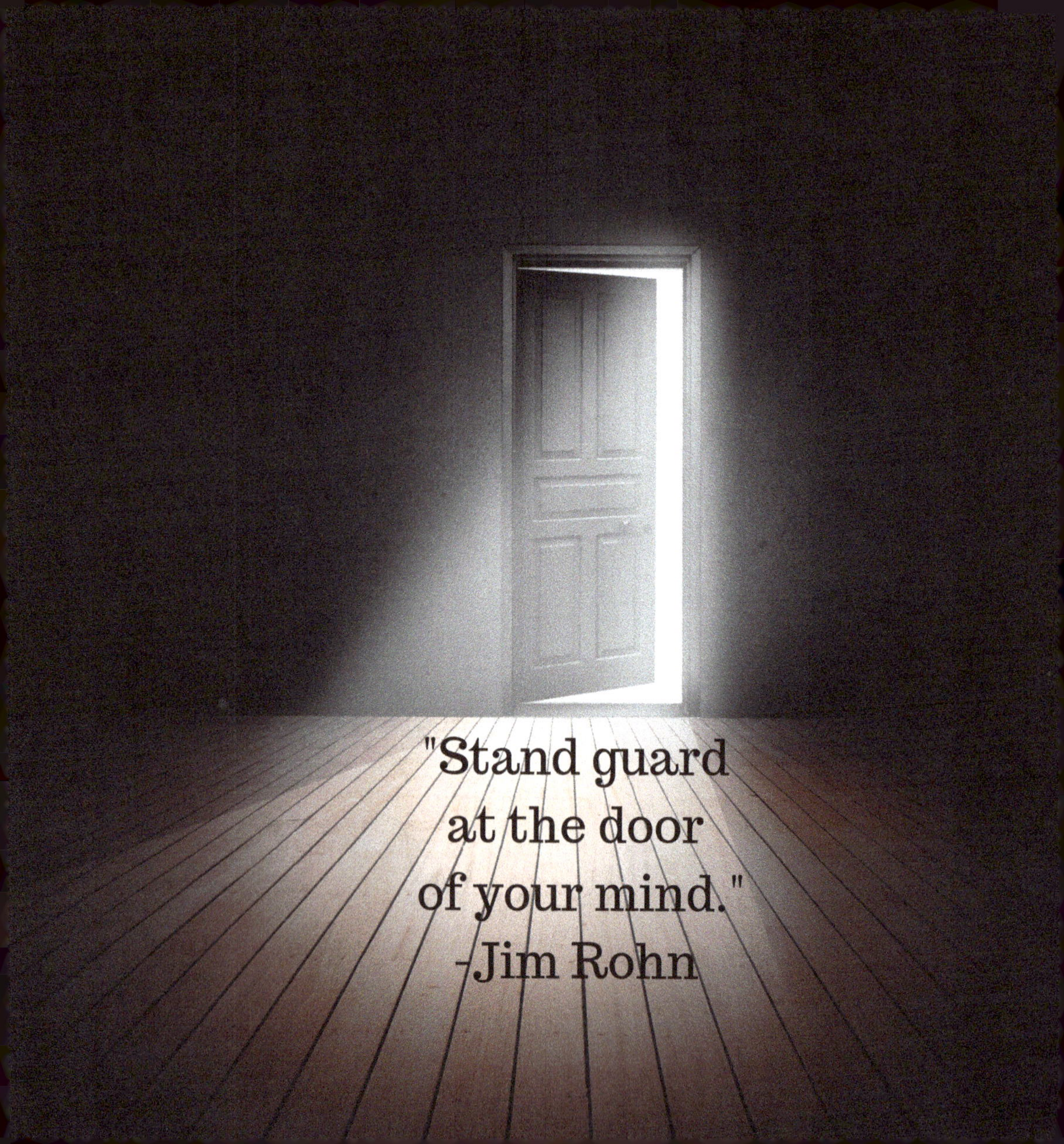

"Stand guard
at the door
of your mind."
-Jim Rohn

Feed your mind with positive input

Just like feeding your body with great nutrition - your mind requires feeding & nurturing as well.
If you don't watch what you let into your mind – negative thoughts from yourself or from others – then you are allowing weeds to grow and spread.

Reduce watching & reading the news, scrolling social media, and being around people who drain you.
Replace this with reading uplifting material, listening to podcasts, watching TED talks, and spending time with people who make you feel great.

Life is a self acceptance path,
not a self improvement path.

-Krishna

Do an excuse detox

Over the next few weeks, catch yourself making excuses and reframe them. These excuses are often about not having enough time, I'm too old, too unfit, not smart enough, not having enough support or money etc.

Instead, focus on what you can do and take ownership of that. Notice how being more accountable empowers you to be more productive increases your focus and creates more energy.

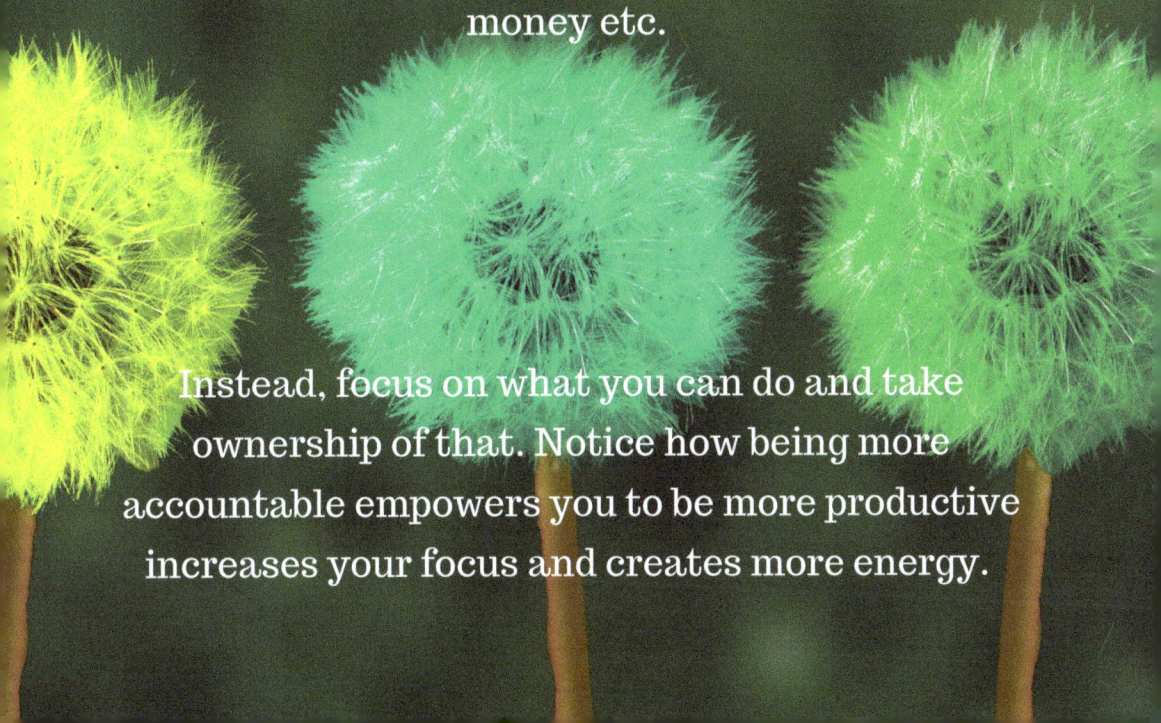

My goal this month is to...

Jan _____

Feb _____

Mar _____

Apr _____

May _____

Jun _____

Jul _____

Aug _____

Sep _____

Oct _____

Nov _____

Dec _____

Tip# 19:

Set a month focused goal

The first of each month is a great opportunity to refocus your life, especially your health & well-being.

Set a focus for the month. It might be:
- drinking more water,
- no snacking between meals,
- being processed sugar-free,
- an alcohol-free month,
- exercise for 20 minutes each morning,
- only push the snooze button once,
- do a short morning meditation,
- learn for 20 minutes each day...

Choose ONE thing and focus on it for the month.

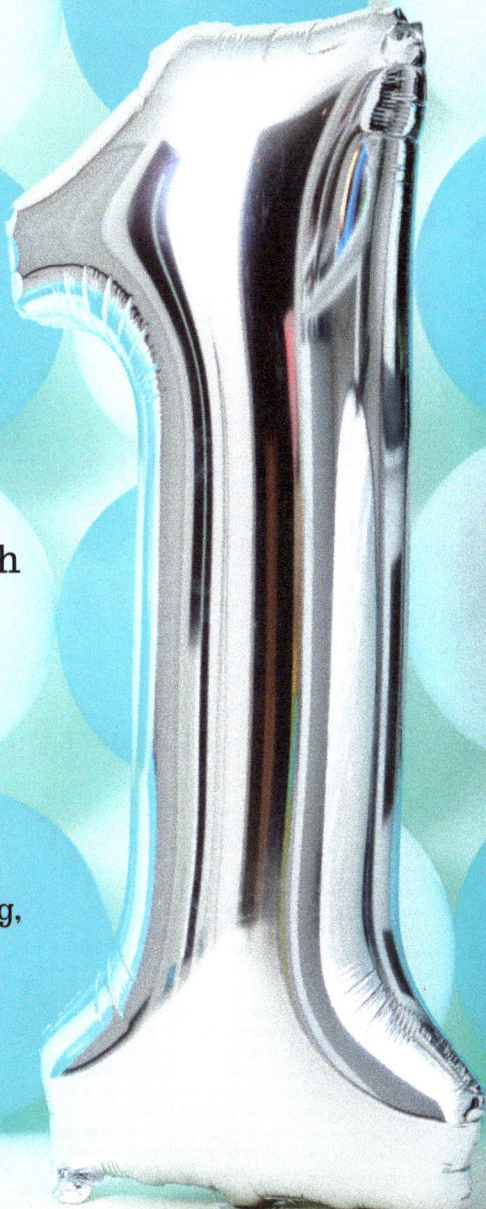

"None of us, including me, ever do great things. But we can all do small things, with great love, and together we can do something wonderful."
-Mother Teresa

Tip# 20:

Encourage your children to help around home

When you work full time, it is important that home is a place of teamwork, rather than feeling like another job. Enrol your children to help around the house. From as young as two years old, children can help with dishes, setting the table, sorting the washing, making their bed, dusting, vacuuming the floors and sweeping the path. It might not be done to the highest standard and it can foster a feeling of inclusion and teamwork and promote less stress.

Focus on what you eat
not on how much you
eat.

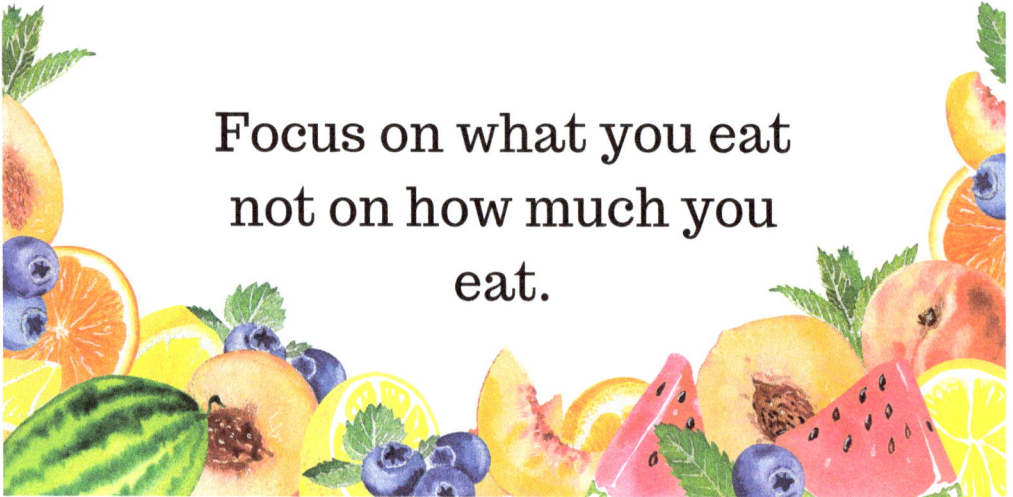

Tip# 21:

Eat nutritious snacks at meetings

Meetings can sometimes lower your energy levels especially when you have had a full day teaching. Provide or bring snacks that will boost and sustain your energy.

Acknowledging the good that you already have in your life is the foundation for all abundance.
- Eckhart Tolle

Tip# 22:

Practice daily gratitude

A regular gratitude practice helps people feel more positive emotions, relish good experiences, improve their health, deal with adversity, and build strong relationships. Create a daily ritual of recalling at least three things you are grateful for. Creating the habit in good times, makes it easier to find gratitude in the harder moments of life.

A book is a gift you can open again and again. - Garrison Keillor

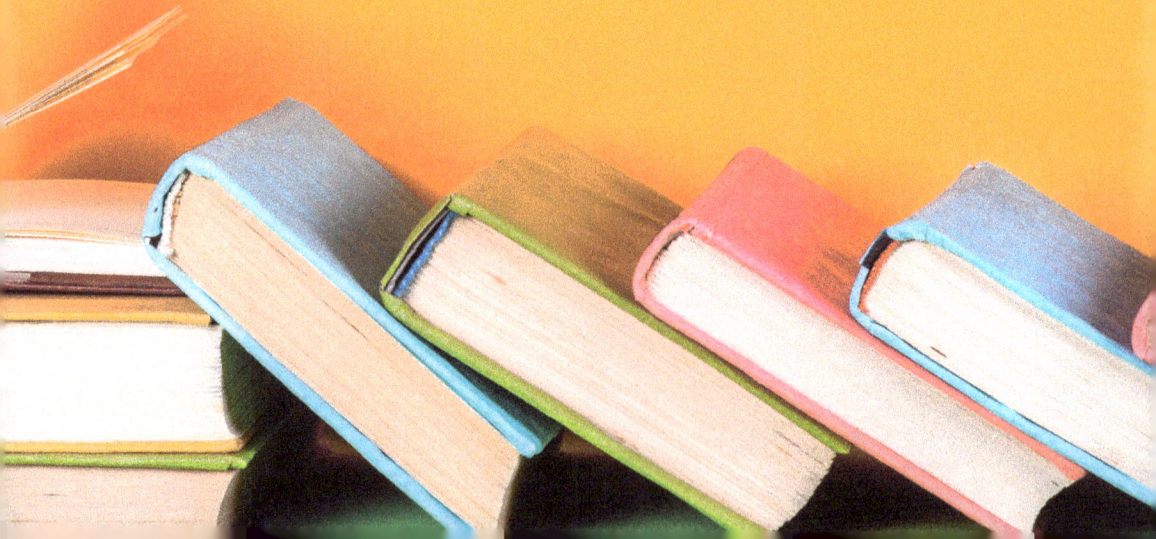

Tip# 23:

Take time to get lost in a book

The benefits of regularly putting time aside to lose yourself in a good book are far-reaching and, in some cases, life-changing. Create time out each day and/or week to read. Just 20 minutes a day reaps positive results. Whether you get lost in a novel, are inspired by a biography, or learning something new, it is good for you. The research shows the benefits of reading include; reducing stress, increasing the quality of sleep, slowing down the onset of dementia and improves your focus and concentration.

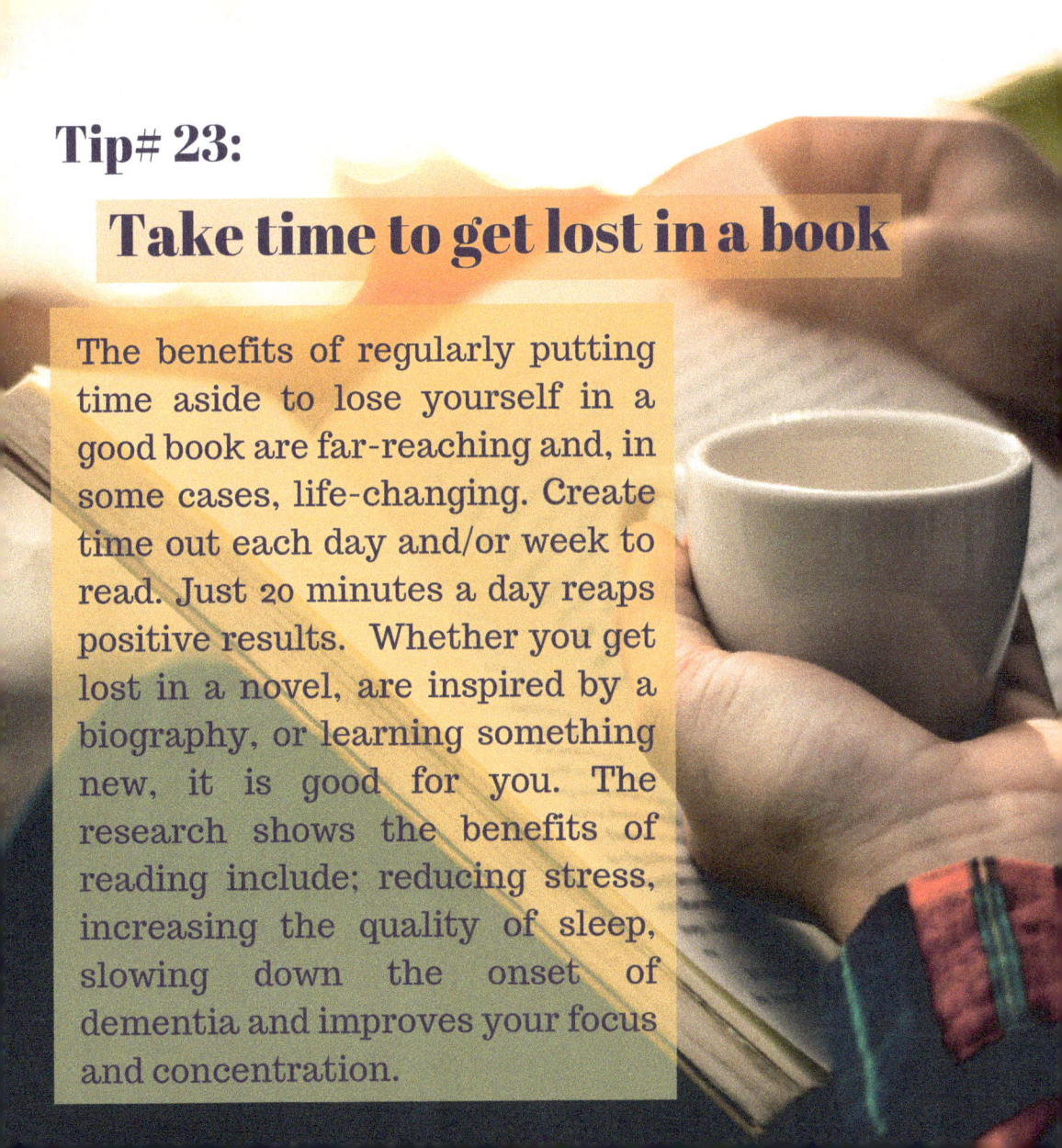

You cannot have a
positive life
and a negative mind.
-Joyce Meyer

Tip# 24:
Reduce negative news

Watching or reading negative news can cause a pessimistic outlook on life. The news is a constant source of negativity that fills our minds with fear and anxiety. These feelings affect your health. Cut out the mass media and focus on your dreams, and goals and making a positive difference in areas you have control over. Reducing negative news can boost your creativity and optimism and ultimately your enjoyment of life.

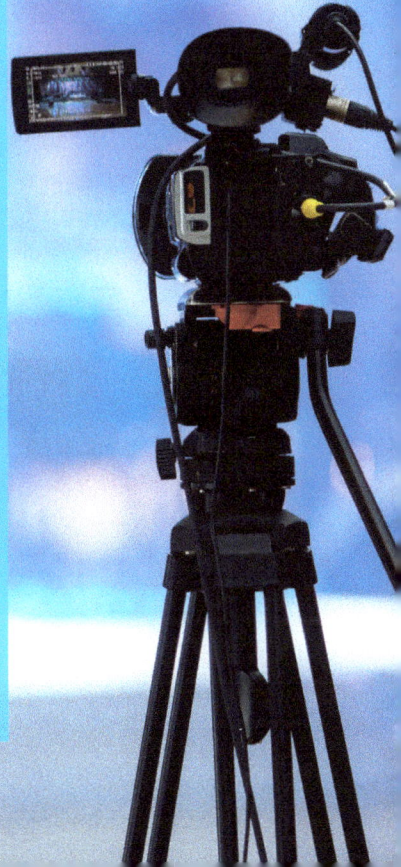

The ability to simplify means eliminating the unnecessary so that the necessary may speak.
-Hans Hoffman

Tip# 25:

Simplify Your Life

Identify what's most important to you and eliminate everything else! Take time to

- evaluate your commitments
- evaluate your time
- simplify work tasks
- simplify home tasks
- learn to say no
- limit your buying habits
- do more of what you love

You can't plan life, but you
can plan dinner.
And that's even better in
some ways.

Simplify your grocery shopping

Type a list of all the items you usually buy at the supermarket and circle when you use something.
Plan your weekly meals to make shopping efficient.
Save time by shopping once a week.
Buy groceries online if available in your area.

"Exercise not only changes your body, it changes your mind, your attitude and your mood."

Tip# 27:

Snack on exercise

Well-being specialist, Lauren Parsons, promotes the value of 'Snacking on Exercise.' She talks about 4 minutes a day - in fact, 4 x 60 seconds each day. Ideas include squats while you wait for the jug to boil, parking further away from the supermarket and taking the stairs.

Good design is as little design as possible.
- Dieter Rams

Minimise your messaging methods

Have you ever gone to look for a message someone has sent you and have to look on several different platforms? Email, text, FaceBook, Messenger, Twitter, Linkedin, What's App, Snapchat - the list goes on. Minimise your messaging methods by choosing 1 or 2 ways people can contact you. This will save you time and energy.

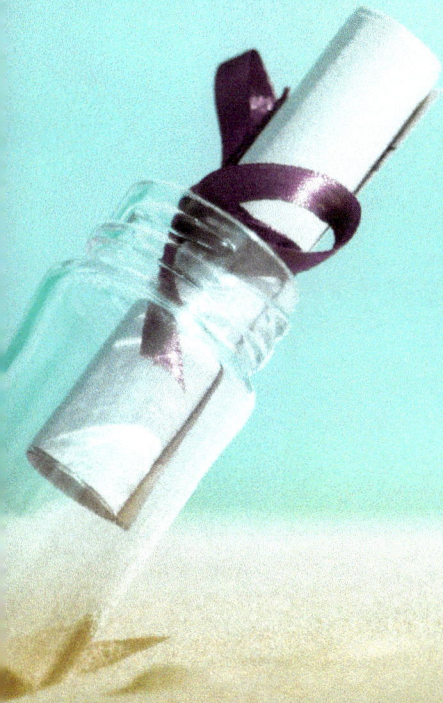

"The minute you start caring about what other people think, is the minute you stop being yourself."
-Meryl Streep

Tip# 29:

Set an energy boost alarm

Boost your energy by setting your phone alarm for 10.30 am and 2.30 pm each day for an energy boost break. Spend one minute boosting your energy.

Ideas include:
- drinking water
- get up from your desk and walking
- run up and down the stairs
- have a dance party
- do some squats, jumps, or skip

Others might think you are crazy - however, they are likely to admire your higher energy and better production levels. Go on just do it!!

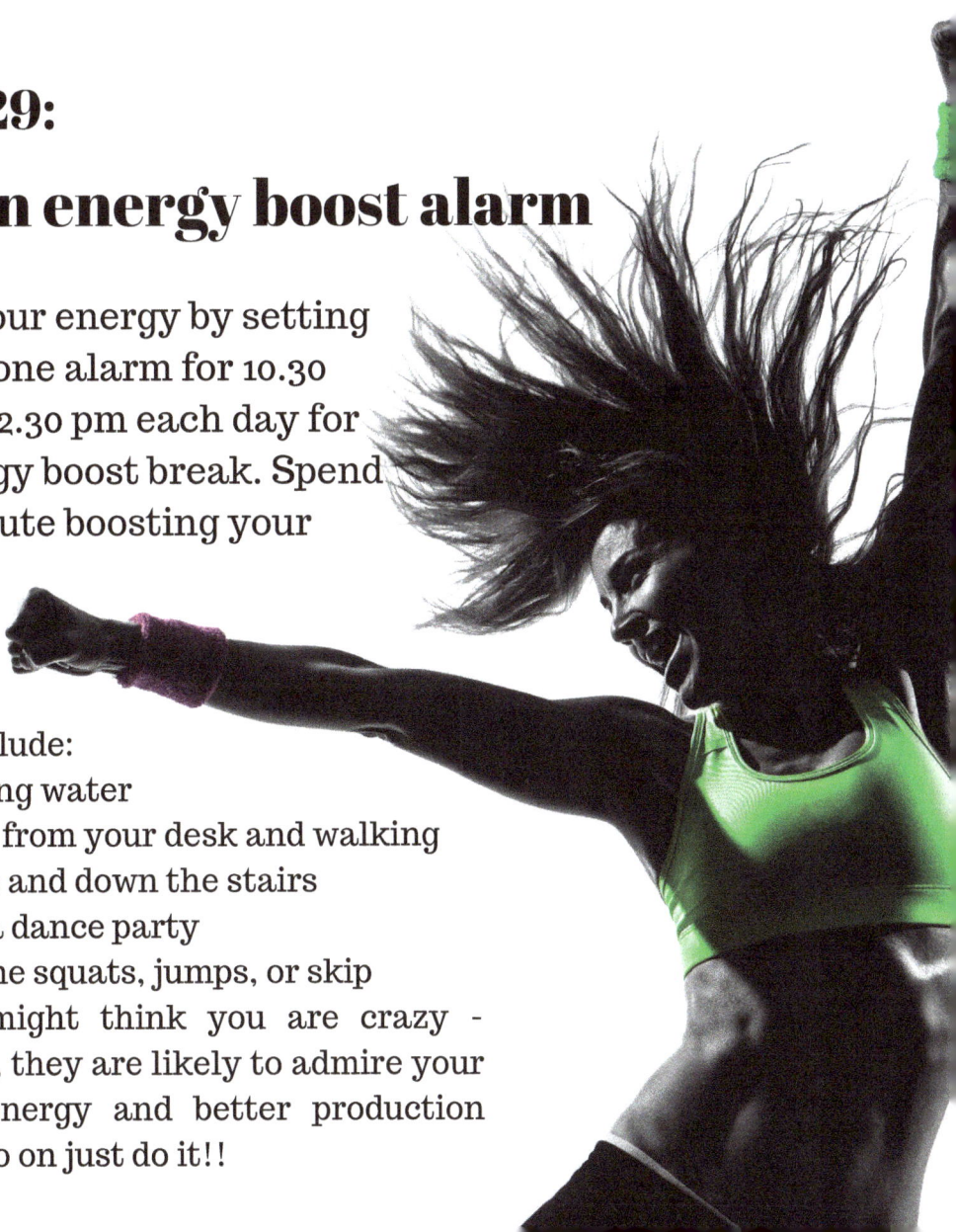

Self love is
consistently
making and then
keeping self
promises
- Robin Sharma

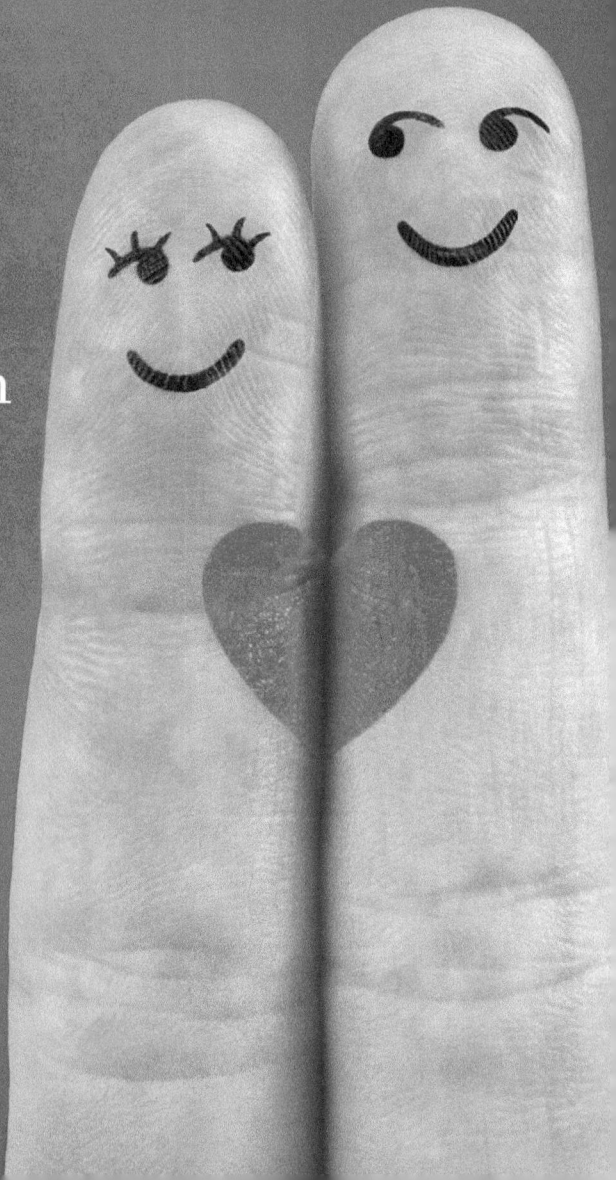

Tip# 30:

What are you doing to stay positive?

Create a morning routine, book some self care, do random acts of kindness, be creative.
Fear cannot exist when you are practising love.

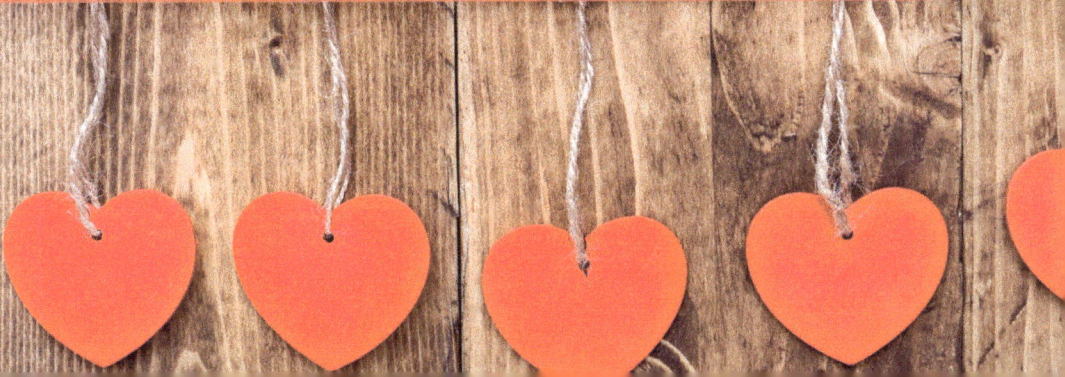

"The best remedy for those who are afraid, lonely, or unhappy is to go outside, somewhere where they can be quite alone with the heavens and nature."
- Anne Frank

Tip# 31:

Spend more time in nature

Studies have shown that being in natural environments can reduce stress, anxiety, and depression while increasing feelings of happiness, calmness, and overall well-being.
Nature can also improve cognitive function, creativity, and attention, as well as boost the immune system and lower blood pressure. Whether it's a walk in the park, a hike in the woods, or a day at the beach, spending time in nature can provide a much-needed escape from the stresses of everyday life and promote a healthier mind and body.

It's not selfish to love yourself, take care of yourself, and make your happiness a priority. It's necessary.
-Mandy Hale

Tip# 32:

Pay for several sessions in advance, buy in bulk or create a monthly payment. This means you have to go for your appointment or self-care treatment.

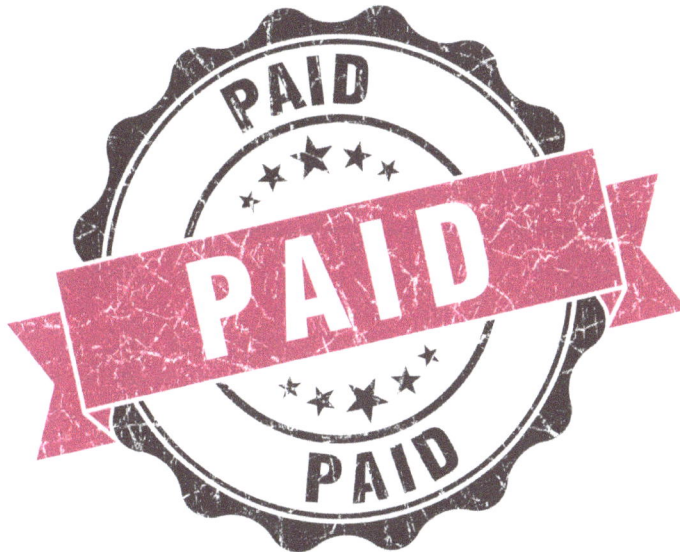

What activities, experiences, things and places bring you joy?

1. _____

2. _____

3. _____

4. _____

5. _____

6. _____

Do more of them!

Tip# 33:

Find
JOY
each day

Take time each day to find or create joy in your life. Maybe ring a friend, light a candle, get out in nature, paint, eat ice cream with sprinkles, laugh, dance, hug the people you love, buy flowers - do something that makes your heart sing.

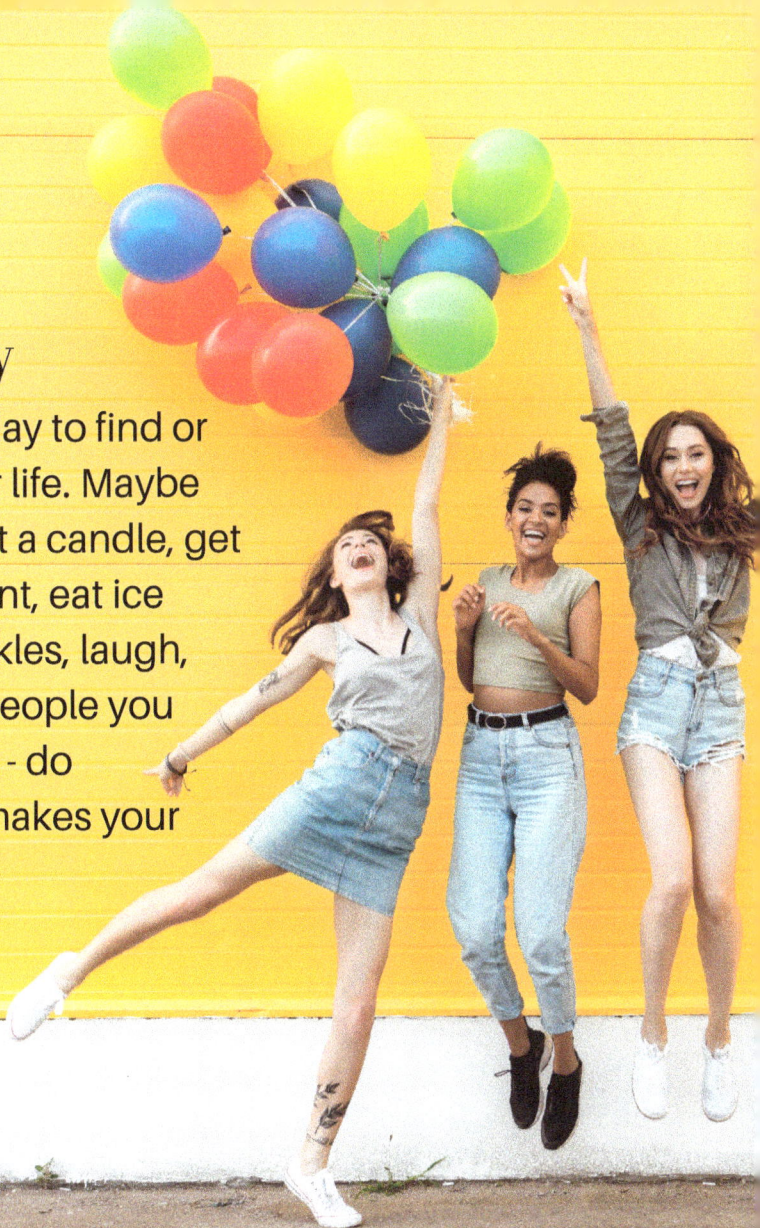

- Start with breath awareness
- Practice mindful eating
- Engage in mindful movement
- Take a mindful pause

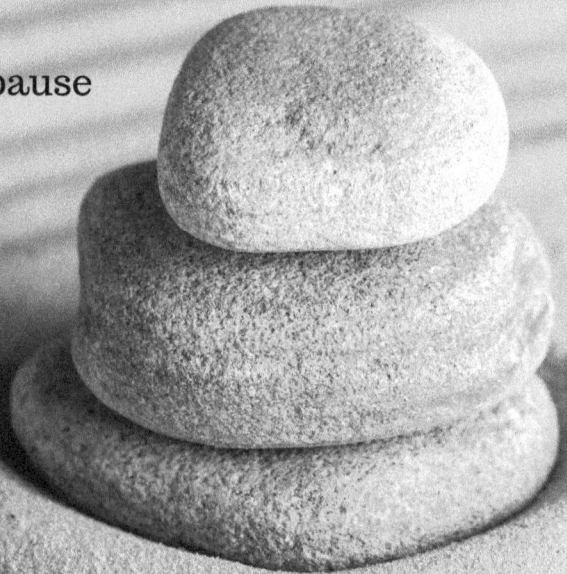

Tip# 33:
Practice Mindfulness

Mindfulness promotes present-moment awareness, non-judgmental acceptance, and emotional regulation It can reduce stress, anxiety and depression, improve concentration and decision-making, and enhance overall mental and physical health. Practising mindfulness can lead to greater self-awareness and a more positive outlook on life.

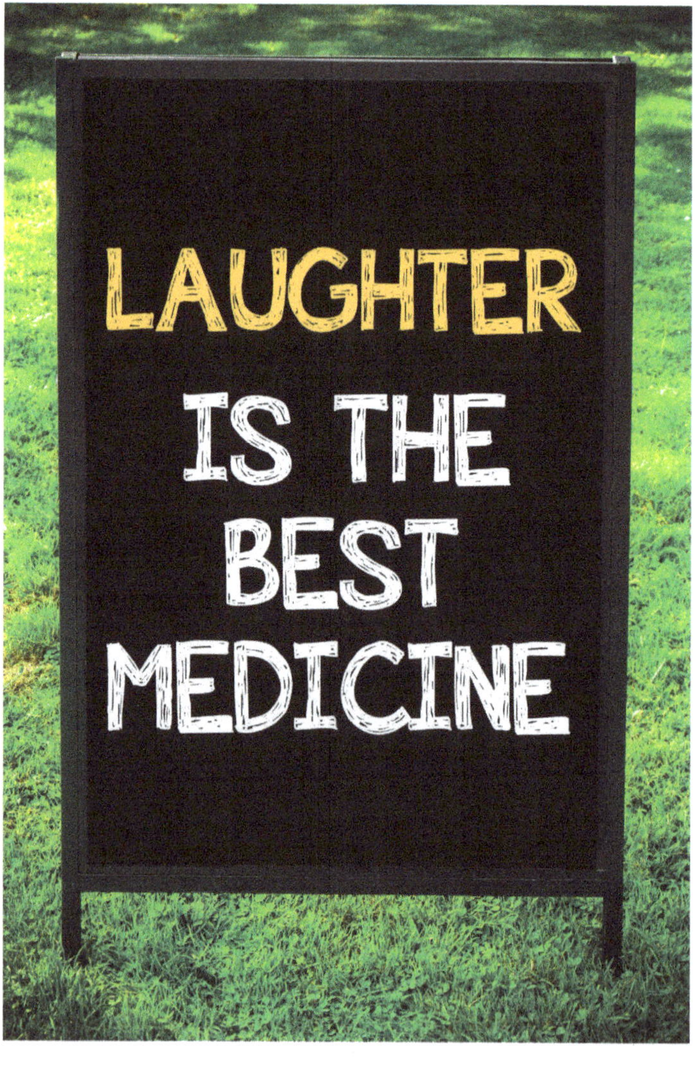
LAUGHTER
IS THE
BEST
MEDICINE

Tip# 34:

Six-year-olds laugh on average
of **600 times a day**.
Adults only laugh **15-100 times a day**.

Be six again

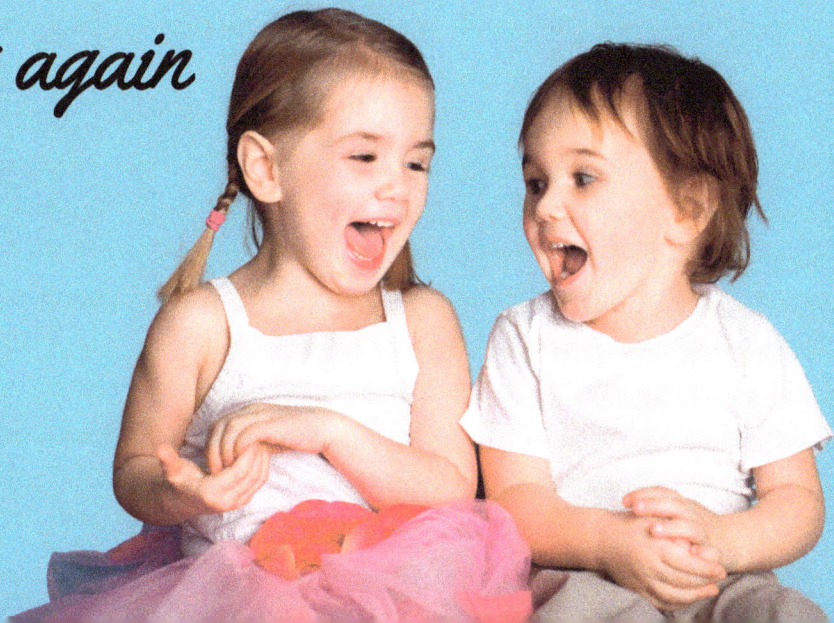

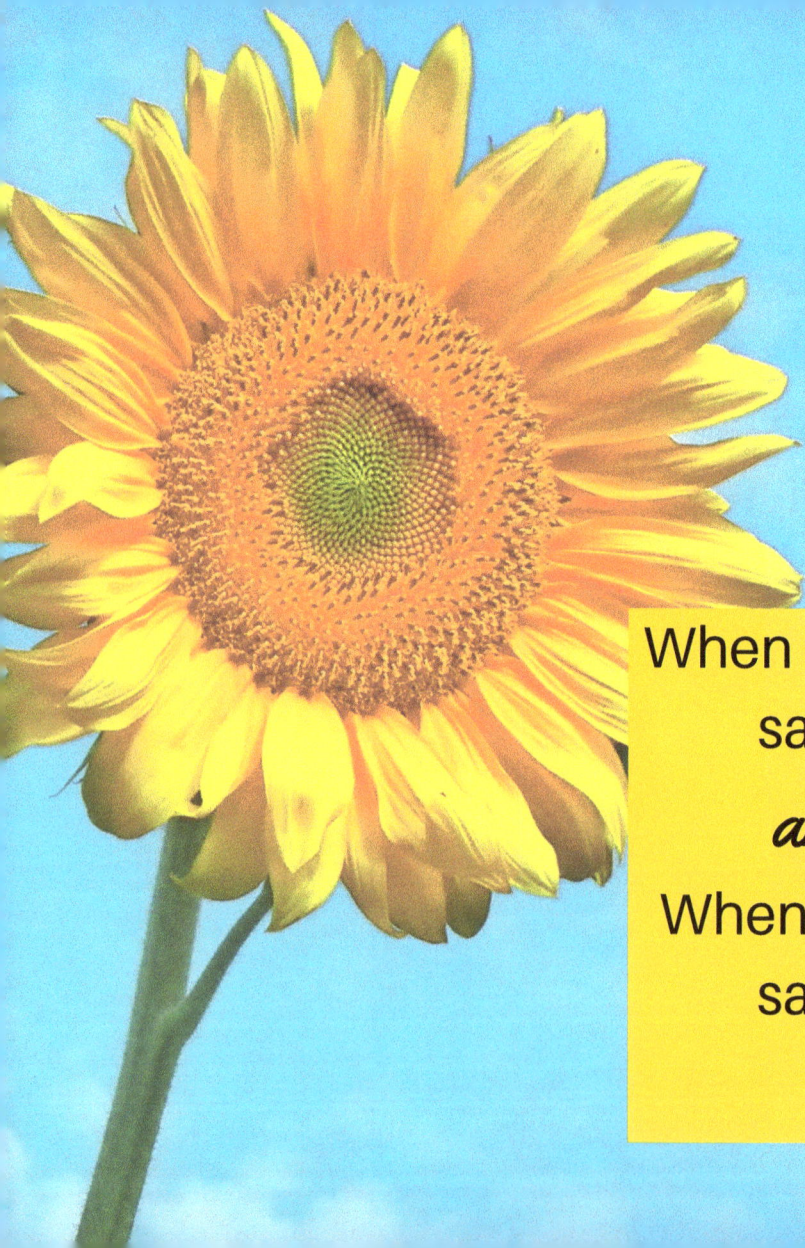

When life is sweet,
say thank you
and celebrate.
When life is bitter,
say thank you
and grow.

About Karen...

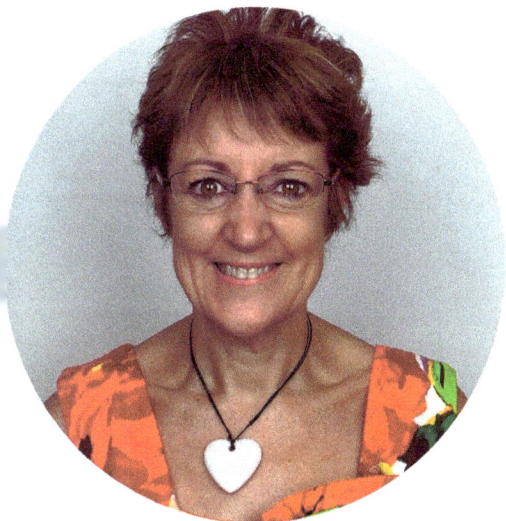

Karen Tui Boyes is a champion for LifeLong Learning. A multi-award-winning speaker, educator and businesswoman, she is an expert in effective teaching, learning, study skills, motivation and positive thinking.

Karen is the CEO of Spectrum Education, Principal of Spectrum Online Academy and the author of 11 books. She loves empowering teachers, parents and students and regularly speaks at conferences and schools. She runs online summits and workshops around the globe and is the wife to one and the mother of two young adults.

Karen was recently named the Global Evolutionary Woman of the Year.

Book Karen for your next PLD day or conference and check out her events and resources at www.spectrumeducation.com.

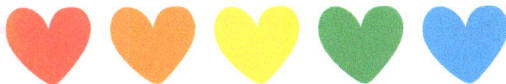

If you do not make time for your wellness - you will have to make time for your illness

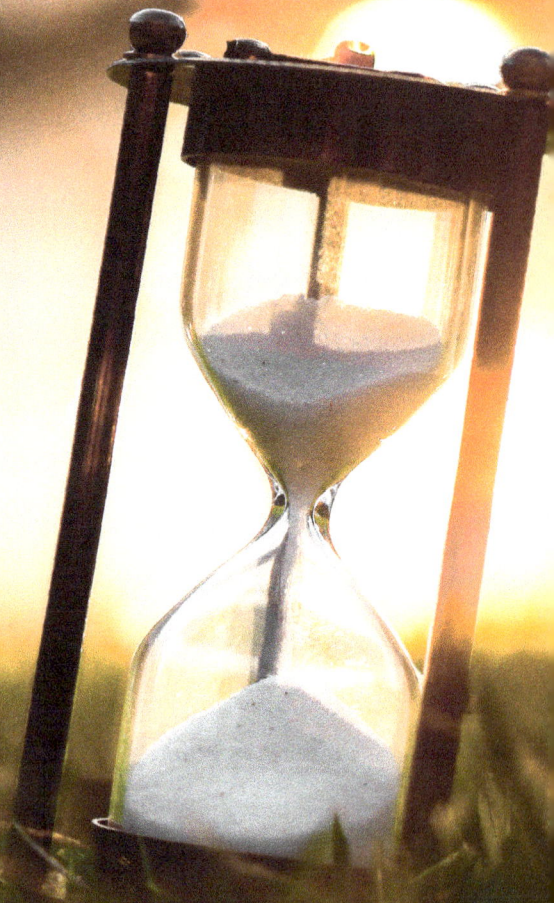

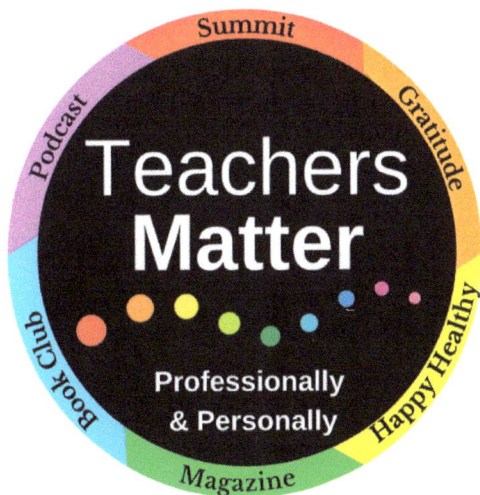

www.ingramcontent.com/pod-product-compliance
Lightning Source LLC
Chambersburg PA
CBHW042357030426
42337CB00029B/5126